Ayurvedic Home Remedies

Natural Remedies to Treat the Most Common Ailments

Contents

Introduction

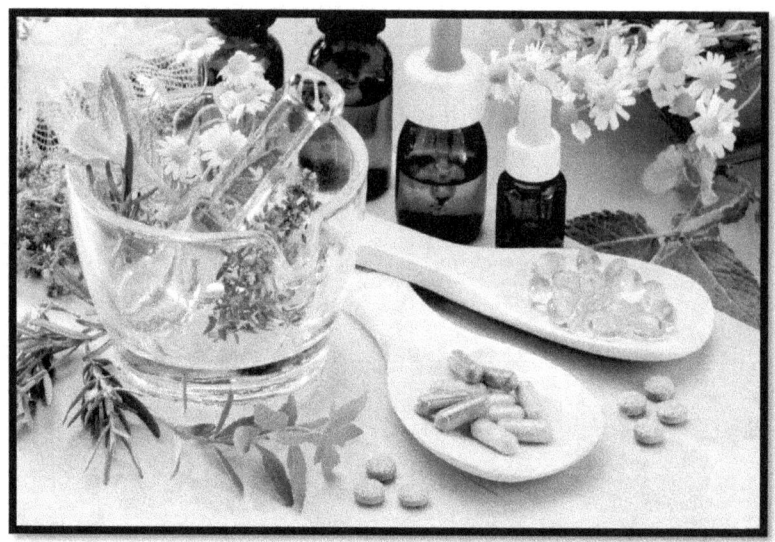

The term "Ayurveda" comes from the Sanskrit term meaning "the science of life." Ayurveda is a system of medicine that has been practiced in India for more than 5,000 years, and it has become an integral part of Indian culture. This type of medicine is similar in its principles and practice to traditional Chinese medicine, but it also incorporates elements of yoga, dietary regulation, detoxification, and certain psychological interventions as well. Simply put, Ayurvedic medicine is an all-natural approach to medicine that aims to not only treat disease but to create balance in one's life and spirit as well.

Not only does Ayurvedic medicine offer treatments for common ailments, but it also places a heavy emphasis on disease prevention. It is believed that maintaining balance in one's mind, body and spirit can help to ensure physical health. The practice of Ayurvedic medicine relies heavily on natural herbs and spices in combination with a healthy diet to prevent and treat disease. In this book, you will receive 20 Ayurvedic remedies for some of the most common ailments including upset stomach, fever, headache, diarrhea, cough and skin problems.

20 Ayurvedic Remedies for Common Ailments

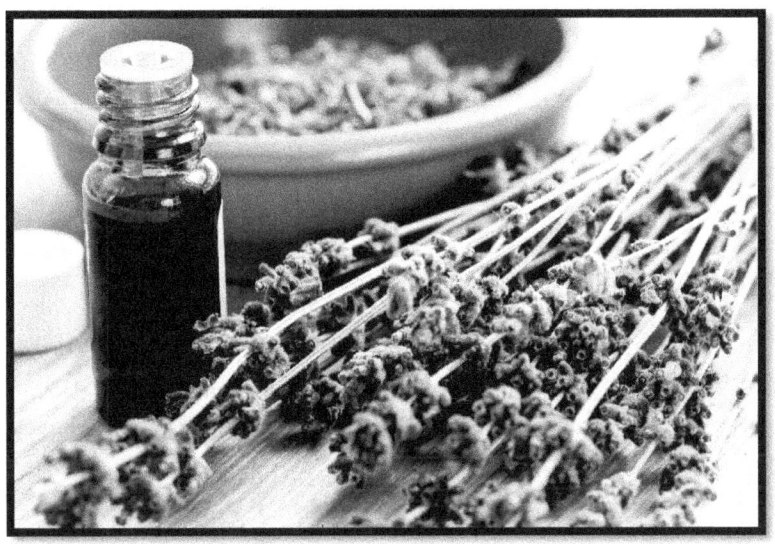

Remedies Included in this Book:

Acne	Cramps	Hair Loss
Anemia	Depression	Indigestion
Asthma	Diarrhea	Insomnia
Chicken Pox	Eczema	Joint Pain
Common Cold	Fatigue	Sore Throat
Constipation	Fever	Stomach Ulcer
Colitis	Flu	

Acne is a condition affecting the skin that is most commonly seen in teenagers – it is caused by excess oil production in the skin glands which leads to blockage of the hair follicles. This condition may present pimples and blackheads and, in severe cases, it can lead to scarring of the skin.

Tips to Restore Balance:

To detoxify your body and improve skin health, try to eat more fresh and wholesome foods. Avoid foods that are spicy, oily, and sour and increase your use of cooling herbs like coriander, fennel and aloe vera. Try to drink at least 8 to 10 glasses of water per day and frequently wash your face with a mild herbal soap.

Ayurvedic Remedies:

1. Combine equal parts coriander seed, dried basil, dried fennel, turmeric, and Indian gooseberry in a small bowl. Grind the ingredients together into a powder and take ½ teaspoon of the powder in liquid 15 minutes before both lunch and dinner.

2. Create a paste using equal amounts of turmeric, saffron, neem, basil, and red sandalwood and a small amount of milk or buttermilk. Apply the paste to your face twice daily and rinse with cool water.

In Ayurvedic medicine, anemia is known as "pandu" and it occurs when levels of red blood cells (RBCs) and hemoglobin fall below normal levels. The normal levels for hemoglobin are 15gm hemoglobin per 100 milliliters of blood and, for RBCs, 5 million red blood cells per cubic milliliter of blood.

Tips to Restore Balance:

Try to follow a well-balanced diet that is rich in protein and fiber. Enjoy foods like sesame seeds, beets, almonds, radish, carrots, tomatoes, bananas and blackberries. You should also try to get at least 15 minutes of sunlight per day because it will help to stimulate the production of red blood cells.

Ayurvedic Remedies:

1. Try taking a cold water bath at least twice per day to control anemia.

2. Enjoy a smoothie made from citrus fruits, apples and beets to increase your body's iron stores which will help to treat the anemia.

In Ayurvedic medicine, asthma is known as "tamak swas," and it is characterized by the chronic but intermittent inflammation of the bronchial airways. This condition may result in episodes of coughing, wheezing and dyspnea.

Tips to Restore Balance:

To avoid aggravating your asthma, try to avoid smoking and limit your exposure to cold or dusty air. Sip warm herbal tea with honey to soothe the throat. Also try to not to eat too much of heavy foods like dairy, fried foods, rice, and beans.

Ayurvedic Remedies:

1. Massage your chest with a mixture of warm sesame oil and salt to loosen phlegm deposits then follow up with a hot shower or steam inhalation.

2. Bring to boil ½ teaspoon of fresh grated ginger in 6 ounces of milk or water then stir in ¼ teaspoon of turmeric. Enjoy this warm tea twice a day.

Chicken pox is a very contagious disease that commonly affects children between the ages of 1 and 10. Symptoms include a rash on the body and face accompanied by small red spots which may develop into blisters. This condition may start with cold-like symptoms with the rash developing one or two days later.

Tips to Restore Balance:

Avoid scratching the rash and bumps as much as possible to reduce the risk for infection. If necessary, make the patient wear gloves or cut their nails short, so they do not open the blisters. In terms of diet, enjoy healthy foods and avoid those that are hard to digest.

Ayurvedic Remedies:

1. Create a paste using sandalwood powder and a few drops of water. Apply the paste to the affected area to soothe itching and irritation.

2. Bring to boil 100 grams of chopped carrot with 60 grams of fresh cilantro (coriander leaves in 500 milliliters of water. Boil the mixture until reduced by half then drink once daily. You may add salt and pepper to taste.

In many cases, the common cold results from weak digestion – when your body doesn't digest food properly, it creates mucus which makes its way into the respiratory system, causing you to cough. A cold can also be the result of allergies or infection of the upper respiratory tract.

Tips to Restore Balance:

Follow a light, warm diet consisting of steamed vegetables and warm vegetable soups. To soothe the throat, enjoy warm herbal teas or hot milk. Avoid all cold foods and drinks as well as sweet fruit juices.

Ayurvedic Remedies:

1. Stir 1 teaspoon fresh ground black pepper and 1 teaspoon of turmeric into 6 to 8 ounces of warm milk and drink once a day.

2. Stir one teaspoon of fresh lemon juice and one teaspoon of honey into a cup of warm water and drink several times daily.

3. Combine equal amounts of ground fenugreek seeds, dried ginger, and turmeric then take 1 teaspoon by mouth in the morning and in the evening.

According to Ayurvedic medicine, constipation is caused by an imbalance of the body energy known as vata. An imbalance of vata results in dryness of the body and causes problems with digestion. Chronic constipation can result in the production of toxins which can spread throughout the body and cause other problems such as arthritis, rheumatism, and high blood pressure.

Tips to Restore Balance:

Engaging in moderate physical activity can help to stimulate healthy digestion. You should also be drinking plenty of water during the day but do avoid drinking water right before a meal. Avoid eating heavy foods as well as foods that are hard to digest – do not eat anything within 2 hours of bed time.

Ayurvedic Remedies:

1. Drink two glasses of water in the morning and gradually increase your consumption to 6 glasses. For the maximum benefit, store your water in a copper container overnight before you drink it.

2. Soak dried figs in hot water overnight then eat them first thing in the morning. You should also drink the water in which they were soaked.

3. Add one teaspoon of fresh lemon juice and a pinch of salt to a cup of warm water. Enjoy this beverage several times per day.

The term "colitis" is used to describe inflammation of the colon and it is caused by chronic inflammation and irritation of the membrane lining the colon. This condition typically starts in the lower portion of the colon and moves upward, causing cramps, abdominal pain, and bloody stool.

Tips to Restore Balance:

Improving your diet is the key to restoring balance and treating colitis. You should begin with a 5-day juice fast to cleanse your digestive tract then follow a diet of small meals of steamed vegetables with rice and yogurt. Juices like cabbage juice and carrot juice are very beneficial but citrus juices should be avoided.

Ayurvedic Remedies:

1. Perform a warm buttermilk enema twice a week to soothe digestive upset and to help reintroduce beneficial bacteria into the colon.

2. Remove the outer skin from 3 or 4 aloe vera leaves and spoon the gel into a small bowl. Combine 3 tablespoons of the aloe vera gel with 6 to 8 ounces of lukewarm water and drink twice a day – once in the morning, once at night.

Muscle cramps are particularly common in adults, but they can occur in children as well. In many cases, muscle cramps are due to poor flexibility and muscle fatigue but they can also be due to dehydration or electrolyte imbalance.

Tips to Restore Balance:

Enjoy foods that are sweet and sour, but avoid dry, cold, and astringent foods. Foods like garlic and vegetables are beneficial. Avoid exposure to cold wind and rain and try a deep tissue massage to relieve cramps and soreness. Try to go to bed early in the evening and incorporate meditation and yoga into your daily routine.

Ayurvedic Remedies:

1. To relieve foot cramps, combine 3 tablespoons of salt with ¼ cup ground ginger and 2/3 cups baking soda in a bucket of warm water. Soak your foot to relax the muscles.

2. For abdominal cramps or gas, combine ¼ teaspoon guduchi with a pinch of shanka brasma and ½ teaspoon of shatavari. Take once or twice daily with food.

3. For other cramps, massage warm sesame oil into the area.

This condition is very common – in fact, it is one of the most common emotional disorders and it can manifest in different ways. Depression results from aggravation of the tama, one of the three vital energies of the mind. In some cases, depression is accompanied by physical symptoms like nausea, headache, constipation, and loss of appetite.

Tips to Restore Balance:

To restore your tama, try to turn your attention away from yourself and to other people or activities. Enjoy moderate exercise to improve both your mental and physical fitness and to promote relaxation. Meditation and yoga may also be beneficial.

Ayurvedic Remedies:

1. Grind up 3 or 4 cardamom seeds and add ½ teaspoon of the powder to a glass of lukewarm water. Stir the mixture then strain it and drink one glass daily.

2. Stir 2 tablespoons of either ashwagandha or brahmi powder into a glass of water and drink twice daily.

3. Crush 5 Indian gooseberries into a paste then strain the mixture to extract as much juice as possible. Stir ½ teaspoon of ground nutmeg into 2 teaspoons of the juice and drink twice daily.

This is a common condition characterized by loose or liquid stools. In many cases, diarrhea is accompanied by abdominal cramps and dehydration – in some cases, it may also present with weakness and a mild fever. Diet is very important for the prevention and treatment of diarrhea.

Tips to Restore Balance:

Avoid eating incompatible foods together like citrus fruits and milk and only eat fried foods in small quantities. Fasting may help the body to flush toxins from the digestive system, but you should not fast if you are already feeling weak. Follow a diet of foods that are easy to digest like yogurt, banana, rice, and apples as well as boiled vegetables.

Ayurvedic Remedies:

1. If you are dehydrated, boil coriander seeds in water and drink frequently. You can also drink pomegranate juice frequently in small amounts.

2. Combine one teaspoon of sugar with ½ teaspoon of salt in 8 ounces of water. Drink this mixture in small doses, about ¼ cup at a time.

3. Make a thick paste using 3 tablespoons of goat's milk and 1 teaspoon of ground sesame seeds and take by mouth.

4. Soak 50 grams of pomegranate skin (fresh) in 800 milliliters of water for 1 hour. Boil the mixture until it is reduced to 25% (about 200ml) then take several tablespoons of the decoction several times daily.

Eczema is a skin condition that results in redness, itching, swelling and dryness as well as a rash that spreads with scratching. In Ayurvedic medicine, this condition is known as "vicharchika" and it is the result of immune system imbalance. This condition is often linked to other allergic conditions.

Tips to Restore Balance:

To avoid irritating your skin, try to wear loose cotton clothing – avoid synthetic fibers because they inhibit perspiration which can further irritate your skin. Use only a mild herbal soap when bathing and dry your skin using a soft towel without rubbing. Avoid oily and spicy foods as well as coffee, tea, and hot spices.

Ayurvedic Remedies:

1. Boil 25 neem leaves in 4 ½ cups of water for a total of 20 minutes. Cool the mixture then use it to bathe the affected area.

2. Combine 1 teaspoon of powdered licorice root with a few teaspoons of warm sesame oil. Apply the oil to the affected area then wrap with a breathable bandage and leave on for 3 to 4 hours. Repeat twice per day.

Fatigue is characterized by a feeling of weariness or tiredness and it can be either chronic or temporary. In many cases, fatigue is the result of poor diet but it can also be caused by various medical conditions including low blood pressure, anemia, infection, or low blood sugar.

Tips to Restore Balance:

Follow a healthy diet and enjoy small snacks of fresh or dried fruit, vegetables, or whole grains between meals. Try to incorporate regular exercise into your routine to relieve tension and to renew energy levels. Alternating cold and hot baths may also help to stimulate your muscles and reduce fatigue.

Ayurvedic Remedies:

1. Stir 1 teaspoon ground licorice root and 2 teaspoons of honey into a glass of warm milk and drink twice daily.

2. Crush 5 Indian gooseberries into a paste (without the seeds) and stir it into 300 milliliters of hot water. Bring the mixture to boil for 20 minutes then cool and strain the liquid. Sweeten with honey, if desired, and drink three times daily.

According to Ayurvedic medicine, fever can be the result of aggravating one, two, or three of the doshas. The symptoms of fever include headache, muscle aches, increased temperature, nausea, and a feeling of heaviness. In some cases, fever is a symptom of another condition like tuberculosis, influenza, or bronchitis.

Tips to Restore Balance:

Your first step to restore balance is to go on a fast to flush toxins and to soothe the aggravated doshas. Follow a diet of easily digested foods including boiled vegetables, fruit juice, and small amounts of cow's milk. Avoid heavy foods and make sure you get plenty of rest.

Ayurvedic Remedies:

1. Create a paste using sandalwood powder and a few drops of water then apply it to the forehead.

2. Combine ½ teaspoon turmeric with 1 teaspoon of honey in a cup of warm milk and drink twice daily.

3. Take 1 teaspoon of fresh lemon juice in a glass of warm water 3 to 4 times daily.

While there are different types of flu, they all have similar symptoms including high fever, cough, sore throat, chills, headache, fatigue and nausea. The flu presents in a very similar way to the common cold but it is typically more severe.

Tips to Restore Balance:

The key to fighting the flu is to bulk up your immune system by getting plenty of rest and by reducing your stress levels. Avoid eating raw, greasy, or overly sweetened foods because this will lead to the stagnation of your Qi which can worsen your flu symptoms.

Ayurvedic Remedies:

1. Combine ½ teaspoon each of ground fennel seeds, ground cinnamon, and ground ginger with a pinch of ground clove in a cup of hot water. Steep the mixture for 10 minutes then strain the tea and drink once daily.

2. Stir 4 grams of ground cinnamon or cloves into a cup of hot water. Let the mixture cool then drink several times daily. You may sweeten the tea with honey, if desired.

3. Stir ½ teaspoon ground turmeric and 2 cloves of crushed garlic into a cup of hot water. Steep for several minutes then strain the mixture and enjoy.

There are many things that can contribute to hair loss including stress, anxiety, and inadequate nutrition. While some amount of hair loss is normal with aging, excess hair loss may be a problem. In Ayurvedic medicine, hair loss is known as "khalitya-paalitya."

Tips to Restore Balance:

Dietary changes can help to restore balance and stop hair loss. Try to avoid spicy or oily foods and do not overindulge in tea and coffee. You should also avoid processed sugars and grains as well as carbonated drinks and alcohol. Eat plenty of fresh fruits and vegetables as well as fresh vegetable juices.

Ayurvedic Remedies:

1. Combine equal amounts of powdered Indian gooseberry and ground sesame seed. Stir 1 teaspoon of the mixture into warm water and drink twice daily.

2. Heat 250 milliliters of coconut oil in a small saucepan and add 4 chopped Indian gooseberries. Cook the berries until they are black then strain the mixture. Massage the oil into your hair two or three times a week.

3. Grind 1 cup of curry leaves with 1 cup of warm buttermilk and apply the mixture to your hair. Let the mixture set for 1 hour then wash your hair with a mild herbal shampoo.

According to Ayurvedic medicine, indigestion causes the production of a harmful substance called "ama". Sleeping during the day can result in indigestion, as can stress, grief, anxiety, and fear.

Tips to Restore Balance:

The key to digesting the "ama" is to fast for two days. After this initial fast, you can follow a diet of fruit and boiled vegetables for a week until the issue is resolved. You can also cook with spices like coriander, cumin, turmeric, ginger, and black pepper.

Ayurvedic Remedies:

1. Sprinkle a slice of raw ginger with table salt and chew it for five minutes before each meal to reduce indigestion.

2. Add ½ teaspoon roasted cumin seeds and a pinch of salt to a glass of warm buttermilk and drink at the end of a meal.

3. Add 1 to 2 teaspoons of fresh lemon juice to a cup of warm water and drink three times daily.

In Ayurvedic medicine, insomnia is known as "anidra" and it involves the inability to fall asleep. Lack of sound sleep has a number of negative impacts on the body and mind and insomnia can be aggravated by several things including stress, lack of relaxation, and improper diet.

Tips to Restore Balance:

To prevent insomnia, try to avoid caffeinated beverages after dusk and do not use your computer or watch television at night. Try a full-body massage with sesame oil followed by a warm bath to promote relaxation and eat foods that are rich in monounsaturated fats like avocado and nuts.

Ayurvedic Remedies:

1. Stir a pinch of green cardamom powder into a glass of warm milk and drink it nightly before bed.

2. Combine 1 teaspoon of ground licorice powder with a glass of milk and drink once in the morning on an empty stomach.

3. Combine 3 grams of fresh mint leaves with 1 cup of water and boil for 15 to 20 minutes. Drink this mixture with 1 teaspoon of honey just before bed.

According to Ayurvedic medicine, joint pain is caused by aggravation of the body energy called vata and accumulation of the energy ama. The ama energy circulates throughout the body and collects in sites of weakness which then aggravates the vata and causes joint pain.

Tips to Restore Balance:

To avoid aggravating joint pain, limit your exercise and avoid exposure to dampness and cold. You can also try massaging your joints with warm coconut oil to improve blood circulation to the area.

Ayurvedic Remedies:

1. Add 1 teaspoon of ground turmeric to a glass of hot milk and drink once daily.

2. Roast ½ cup of fenugreek seeds then crush them into a fine powder. Combine 2 teaspoons of this powder with a few drops of water to make a thick paste then apply the paste to the affected area.

3. Soak 3 tablespoons of green gram in 250 milliliters of water overnight then stir 2 minced garlic cloves into the mixture. Consume this mixture twice daily.

Sore throats are commonly connected to colds and flu and they typically cause pain, inflammation, and irritation of the throat. In some cases, the neck may become tender and swollen and the back of the throat may redden and become covered in a gray or whitish mucus.

Tips to Restore Balance:

Begin with a fast of orange juice and water for 3 to 5 days. Once the most severe symptoms go away, introduce fruit to the diet for another 3 or 4 days. You may then adopt a normal diet that is heavy on nuts, seeds, whole grains, fresh fruit, and raw vegetables.

Ayurvedic Remedies:

1. Add ½ teaspoon freshly ground black pepper, ½ teaspoon ground cinnamon, and ½ teaspoon salt to 8 ounces of hot water. Let the mixture cool then gargle with it twice daily.

2. Combine 1 tablespoon fresh lemon juice with ½ teaspoon ground black pepper and ½ teaspoon salt. Heat the mixture slightly then drink once daily.

3. Bring a 1-inch piece of peeled ginger with 6 to 8 ounces of water to boil for 2 to 3 minutes. Sweeten with honey, if desired, and drink several times daily.

Stomach ulcers occur when the lining of the stomach becomes less resistant to acids and digestive juices. In Ayurvedic medicine, a stomach ulcer is known as "annadravshool" and an ulcer of the duodenum is called "parinaamshool." Ulcers typically cause pain in the chest after eating.

Tips to Restore Balance:

Limit your diet to light, easy-to-digest foods and avoid any heavy, spicy, or sour foods that could aggravate the ulcer. Enjoy brown rice or parboiled rice as well as coconut water, barley water, whole-wheat flour, and cow's milk. Avoid fasting because having an empty stomach can aggravate the ulcer.

Ayurvedic Remedies:

1. Combine 1 teaspoon of unrefined sugar with a pinch of green cardamom powder in a glass of cold milk. Drink this mixture whenever you have pain, or 3 to 4 times daily.

2. Combine ½ teaspoon unrefined sugar with 1 teaspoon of Indian gooseberry powder and enjoy twice daily on an empty stomach.

3. Combine 1 teaspoon unrefined sugar with 1 teaspoon roasted barley flour in a glass of water and enjoy 3 to 4 times daily.

Conclusion

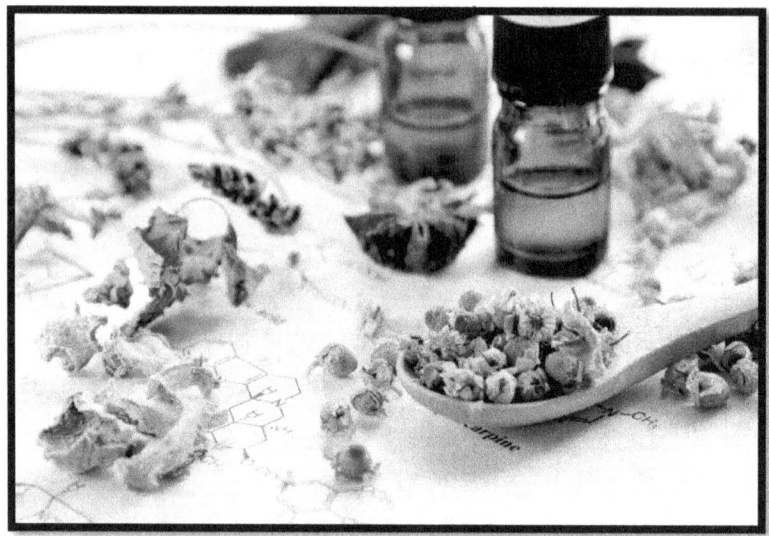

      In reading this book, you have learned not only the basics regarding what Ayurvedic medicine is but also what it can do for you. Similar to traditional Chinese medicine, Ayurvedic medicine incorporates a number of different elements of health and wellness to ensure balance of both the mind and spirit. According to Ayurvedic principles, imbalance is the cause of disease so treatments are designed to restore balance. Many common ailments including skin problems, joint problems, and gastrointestinal issues can be remedied using Ayurvedic medicine. If you are ready to see what Ayurvedic medicine can do for you, simply give one of the remedies in this book a try – you may be surprised at how well it works!